Skin Care Made Simple... Toning Tips for Women of All Ages

Teaching Women of Any Age Proven Methods to Maintain Healthy and Radiant Skin Tone

Terms and Conditions
LEGAL NOTICE

Table Of Contents

Foreword

If you're anything like me, you can be completely overwhelmed by the amount of various skin care products out there. So, becoming more and more confused by the onslaught of potions and lotions, I decided to take the appropriate journey to figure the best method and applications needed for myself and others.

I have daughter's that are in their late teens and early 20's. Without any question, helping them was at the top of my priority list. Of course they have always looked to me for guidance, so my journey toward understanding what they needed for their skin was of extreme importance to me.

And it didn't end there. I have good friends in their 30's and 40's. Their needs are very specific, and it became a personal mission (as I am in that age group), to find out what could be done to give them the best advice. Finding out the best products and how to use them accentuated our friendships, and enabled them to have much better results in their quest to look and feel better about themselves.

Certainly the need for younger looking skin becomes even more important for women moving into their later years. My efforts for the two previous age groups uncovered many ways to achieve younger looking skin, greatly reducing wrinkles and the dreaded dark spots and blemishes. It has been a distinct pleasure to be able to have any woman thank me for helping them look and feel younger, but especially when it comes to women who are moving into or are into their senior years.

This book is simply one woman's outlook on what works best in my world, and I wanted to share that with you.

Introduction

This is an article about skincare. I have brought this together from my own point of view. In this book, I would like to try and explain why skincare is important and how you may like to introduce, think about, or modify your present skincare routine.

The skin is continually repairing and renewing itself. When you are young, the main skin complaints are greasy skin and acne. But as you grow older, the skin gets dry and the challenge is how to address the dryness of the skin. However, you can have beautiful skin no matter what your age, race or color. The secret is to understand how your skin functions, and to take care of it properly.

The Skin is composed of cells, sweat pores, and sebaceous glands. The surface layer of the skin is covered with a thin sheath of dead cells. These are continually being pushed up to the surface from below. If the dead cells are not removed, they can reduce and even block the skin's effort to breathe and eliminate waste.

For most of us, when we refer to skin care, we mean caring for the face. It is true that the face, usually more than any other part of the body, needs care and attention. The face is constantly exposed to the elements, even in severe winter when the rest of the body is well wrapped. Hence, the face is one of the first parts of the body to show signs of aging.

Most soaps remove the natural oils of the skin, change the natural pH levels and do nothing to remove the dead layers of skin, which can block your pores and lead to blackheads. The skin produces oils and acids to help it function, to protect it from loss of excessive moisture and to form a barrier.

Chapter 1 Exfoliating Skin

Exfoliation itself is essential for skin health ,and most skin types can benefit from exfoliation.WHO CAN EXFOLIATE THEIR SKIN? Any gender, any age. And all skin types, from dry skin, oily skin, skin with blackheads, acne, sun-damaged skin, flaky skin, etc. The goal is to use the most effective product for exfoliating skin. Using an exfoliate steps in to help put everything in balance again. When you gently get rid of built-up skin cells you can undo clogged pores, stop breakouts, smooth out wrinkles, even make dry skin become a thing of the past! Apply a moisturizing cream immediately after exfoliation.

This process may produce some redness, which will go away within a few hours. People who are prone to redness should exfoliate at night, giving their skin time to calm while they sleep. If you have extremely dry skin, apply a thin coat of moisturizing oil 5 minutes prior to exfoliation.

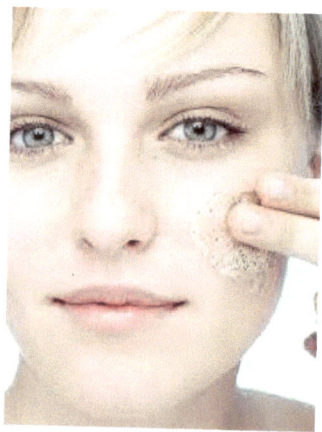

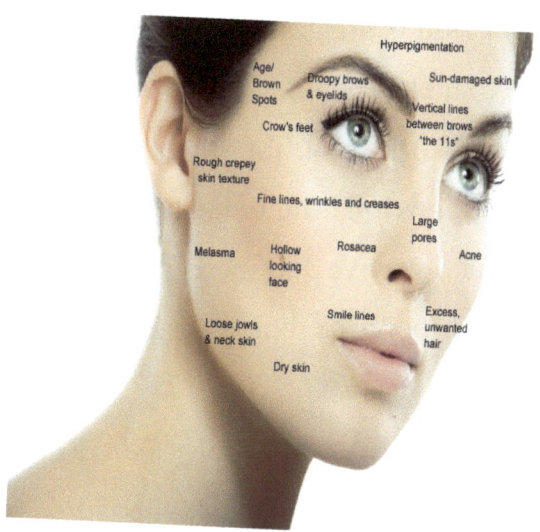

Exfoliating Can Make You Look Instantly Younger

How is that possible? Think about it in comparison to the skin on your heels before you get a pedicure. The built-up, dead layers of skin on your heels usually looks dry, scaly, and lines are really obvious. Once that layer is removed, your heels immediately look smooth and unwrinkled! Of course, what causes calluses on your feet is different than what causes skin cells to build up on your face, but the same benefit of exfoliating heels holds true for your face; you just have to be far gentler.

Is it Possible to Exfoliate Too Often?

Exfoliating your skin is great, but how often to use one that works best for your skin type takes experimenting. For some people once a day works best, for others every other day, or once a week. If anything, exfoliating unhealthy dead skin cells on the surface of skin can improve and increase the skin's ability to hold moisture, and allow pores to function normally.

Exfoliation is essential to good healthy skin. The skin is essentially the largest part of your body, and treating it properly will ensure not only a better look, but afford you with a better and healther complexion. Treating your skin and exfoliating in the ways described here will bring you many years of looking and feeling great!

Chapter 2   Facial Mask

Face masks are the perfect skin care treatment to help you with your skin care concerns. The right face mask can help hydrate skin, remove excess oils and help improve the appearance of your pores. They're also an excellent way to help pull out impurities. Another advantage of wearing a face mask: the feeling of being pampered like you're at a spa from the comfort of your own home!

You can use a face mask once a week, or you can use it more often depending on your skin type and your specific skin care concerns to bring out the skin's healthy radiance. Face masks don't just offer results that improve the overall appearance of your skin, they can also be quite therapeutic.

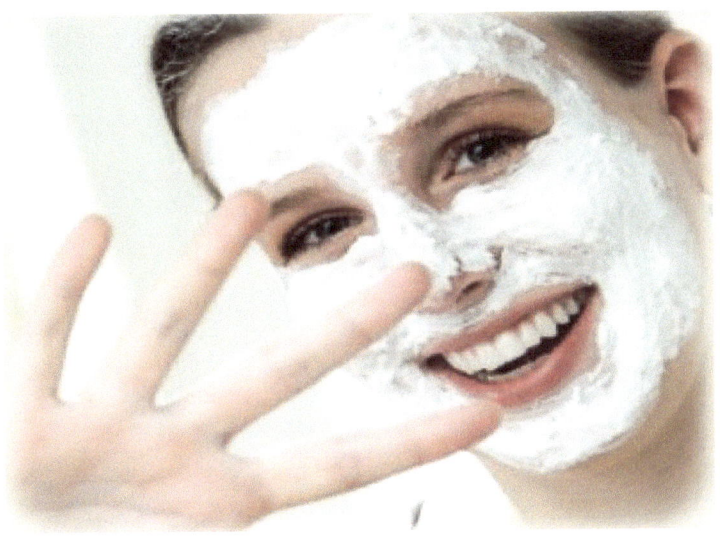

Masking helps all of your other skin care products work more efficiently. If you want your day lotions, serums and nighttime products to be absorbed by your skin quicker and deeper, then a face mask is a must. By masking on a regular basis, you can ensure that your toning, hydrating and protecting products will all perform better, allowing you to achieve much quicker results.

Only a good facial mask can help to draw out impurities that hide beneath the top layers of the epidermis. Some people say that their skin goes through a "detoxing" when they use a mask because they actually notice the changes in the skin while this is happening.

Masks are incredible at providing this deeper cleansing process, leading to an improvement in the appearance of pores that you can see and feel. Who doesn't love that?

Chapter 3 Excessively Oily Skin Solutions

Oily skin occurs when glands produce a high level of sebum (oil) on the skin. Often, people with oily skin have large pores, and are prone to acne as well as shiny skin. But if you have oily skin, don't worry too much about it, as having naturally oily skin is less prone to wrinkles than dry skin. The oil keeps skin moist, which keeps wrinkles away, and is a good thing!

Oily skin could also be due to hormonal changes (which are most often seen in a person's teens/early 20s). You could also have combination skin – meaning that some areas of your face are oily, and some are dry.

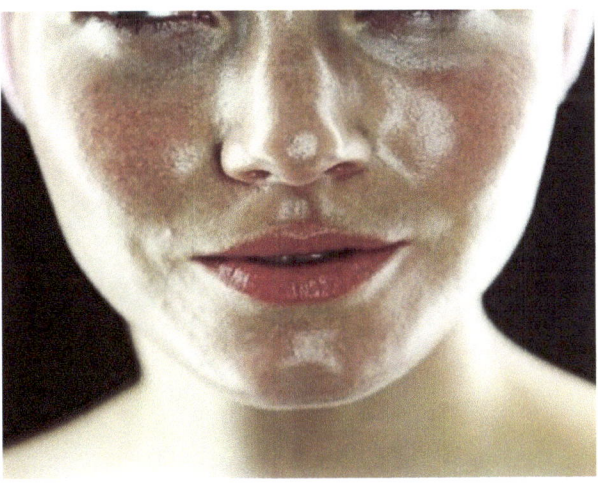

Five steps to keep oily skin under control

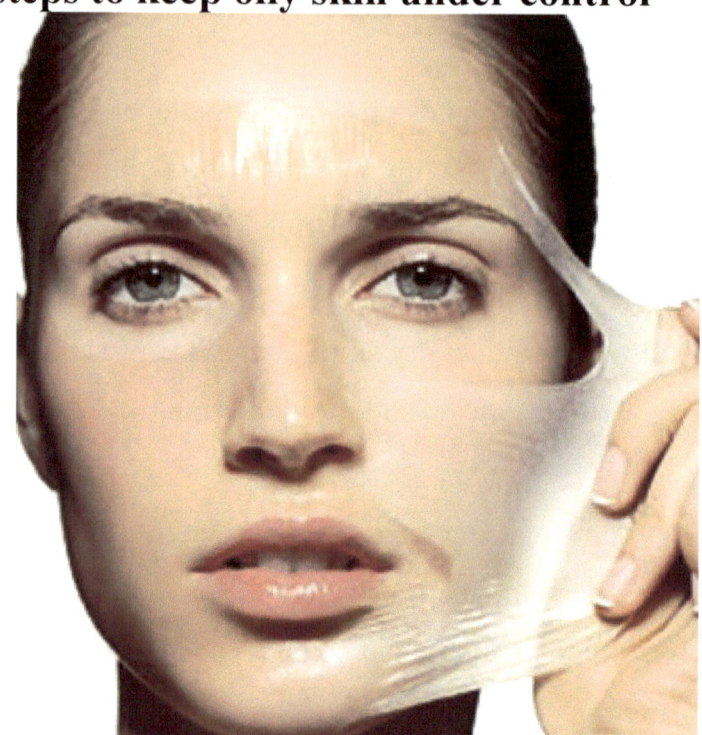

1. Always carry oil blotting sheets and tissues, which help you control shine throughout your day. Oil blotting sheets are an inexpensive way to mop up excess oil on your face and give you a matte look for hours after you've cleansed your face.

2. If you use cosmetics, look for those that are oil-free or water-based. You could use **Silica**, which is an oil absorber helping to absorb excess oils that may be present.

3. Or you could try **Willow Bark Extract,** which is a toning agent that is known to provide mild astringents that won't allow for excess oil production. What could be better for matte makeup?

4. Try different moisturizers. Sometimes oily skin is only present in certain areas of the face such as the T-zone (the t-shaped zone of your forehead, nose, and chin), but cheeks are still considered dry or normal. The areas of your face that are oily may need a lighter moisturizer, so keep trying moisturizers until you find the one that is perfect for you.

5. Pull your hair back. Although hair can be beautiful when you leave it down, it can also exacerbate oily skin. If you have oily skin, try to keep your hair out of your face as much as possible to prevent clogged pores and excess shine.

6. Make skin care a ritual. Good skin starts with good habits. If you have oily skin, consider adding an extra step to your beauty routine masks. Clay masks are great for removing impurities and decreasing the visibility of the pores.

Chapter 4 Skin Tips for Today's Women

Today's women put skin care at the top of their beauty preparation. If you're not using a cleanser, moisturizer or day/night solution in your everyday life style, you are missing out on having rejuvenated skin.Adding a good exfoliating product to your routine once a week will help prevent the pours from clogging up with built-up skin cells. Don't have time for intensive skin care? You can still pamper yourself by doing the basics.

Choose a moisturizer that matches your particular skin type. For example, you may need a thick cream for extremely dry skin or a gentle formula for sensitive skin. For the daytime, use a moisturizer with a built-in sunscreen of SPF 35.

Good skin care and healthy lifestyle choices can help delay the natural aging process and prevent various skin problems. Healthy skin is the key to a youthful looking complexion. So begin with these simple steps to have a healthier skin tone.

1. Cleanser
2. Microdermabrasion twice a week
3. Facial Mask twice week
4. Moisturizer
5. Day sunscreen SPF 35 / Night solution

Chapter 5   Managing Dark Spots and Blemishes

Dark spots on the skin are typically caused by sun damage or the skin being exposed to excess sunlight.   If that area has somehow been damaged previously, these dark spots or blemishes occur much more quickly. Hormonal imbalances, like those associated with pregnancy, can trigger this over-pigmentation of the cells. In addition, as people age, the skin may not reproduce as easily. This can make it more difficult for the skin to heal itself and eliminate those dark spots. Acne can also create scars leaving dark spots or blemishes on the skin.

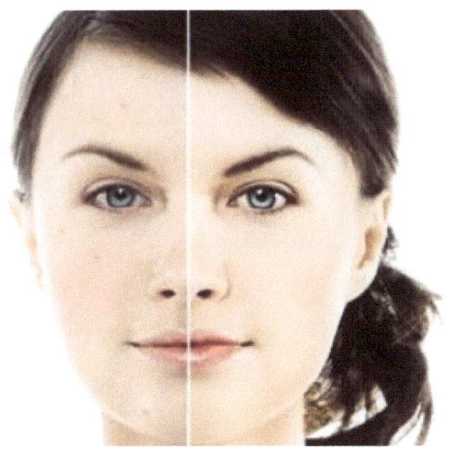

The key to addressing these issues is to find as many dark "erasers" as possible. Vitamin E applied externally and additional intake of vitamin C will help.

In addition, external applications of pineapple, honey, horseradish, yogurt, cucumber, potato, turmeric, and papaya are very effective. You need to leave those applications on the skin for a few minutes to aid in the reducing or removal of the dark spots.

My personal favorite remedies are below

My Most Effective Dark "Erasers"

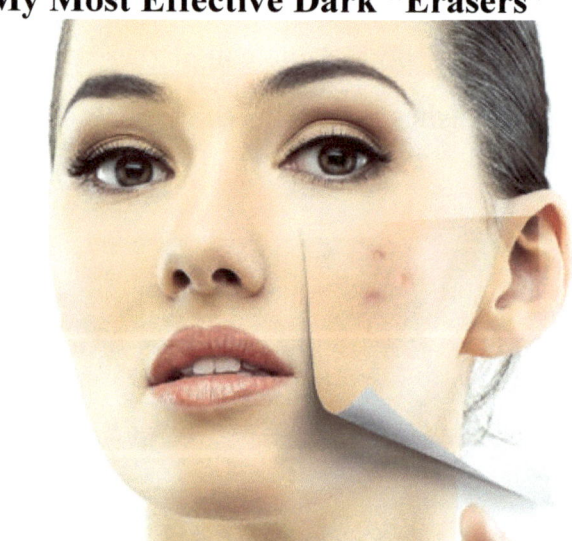

Cleanser : Cleansers help to remove all of the dirt, oil and other impurities from skin. Women, removing makeup is an absolute must, and even more so as we enter our twenties.

Masks that contain : Sunflower oil, omega-6 ,antioxidant acid,vitamin C, Plum Extract

Moisturizer Essence: Lucentrix complex is known to provide a brightening effect, resulting in more even-looking skin.

Microdermabrasion;

Microdermabrasion therapy uses microscopic crystal particles to remove layers of damaged skin, allowing new, fresh skin to be seen.

Sunscreen Cream;

Wearing sunscreen cream every time you go outside, even in colder months, can help prevent sun spots from forming on the skin. Put sunscreen cream generously on the face around 30 minutes before going outside so it has a chance to take effect.

Chapter 6   Managing Acne Problems

Acne occurs when the pores of your skin become clogged, most often on the face, neck. Once a pore becomes clogged, it traps skin oil inside. Bacteria grows in this oil and can cause an inflammatory response in the skin. Acne can be small and hardly noticeable, have a small white or black head, or can appear red with a white/yellow center.

Men and women both suffer from breakouts, and I can assure you that nobody is thrilled when it happens. Everyone—men and women alike, must cleanse their face every single day. Facial cleansing is a must, and should be done in the morning and the evening before bedtime. Choose a cleanser that is most appropriate for your skin type. If you have frequent breakouts, your skin is probably on the oily side, so choose a gel-based cleanser that will help control and remove sebum from the skin.

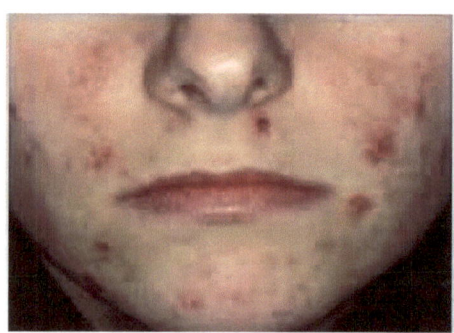 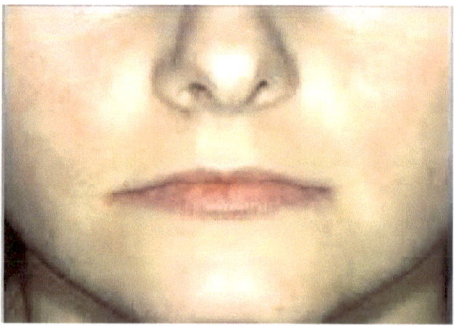

You can reduce your acne by following these skin care tips:

1. Wash twice a day and after sweating. Wearing a hat or helmet can make acne worse, so wash your skin as soon as you remove them. Those sweat glands, though critical to bodily function, must be kept clean to avoid the acne issue.

2. Use your fingertips to apply a gentle, non-abrasive cleanser. Using a washcloth, mesh sponge or anything else can irritate the skin.

3. Be gentle with your skin. Use gentle products, such as those that are alcohol-free.

4. Rinse with lukewarm water.

5. Let your skin heal naturally. If you pick, pop or squeeze your acne, your skin will take longer to clear and you increase the risk of getting acne scars.

The Fact Is

There is no other oral treatment for acne which produces long lasting remission of acne symptoms. However, the proper ongoing treatment can get the skin completely clear, and keep it that way for years. Treatment that has   fragrance-free, oil-free, non-comedogenic, and that is suitable for sensitive skin would be the way to for best results.

Chapter 7 Facial Cleansing Brush For Soft, Clear Skin

There are so many benefits from using an exfoliating brush on your face, everyone should own a face brush and use it regularly. Two speed settings allow you to customize the intensity of your cleansing experience. Waterproof* for use at the sink, shower or bath would be recommended.

Here are a few of tricks for cleansing-brush rookies:

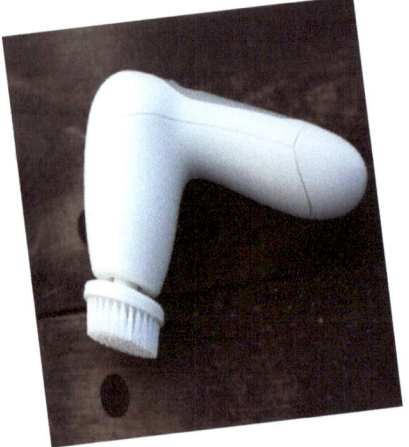

Start using a face wash with acne treatments such as a salicylic or glycolic   acid before you use your brush for the first time as a preventative measure.

Ease the brush into your routine. Try using it once or twice a week at first and slowly build up your use.

Follow up your cleansing with any topical medications you may use, then with moisturizer and SPF.

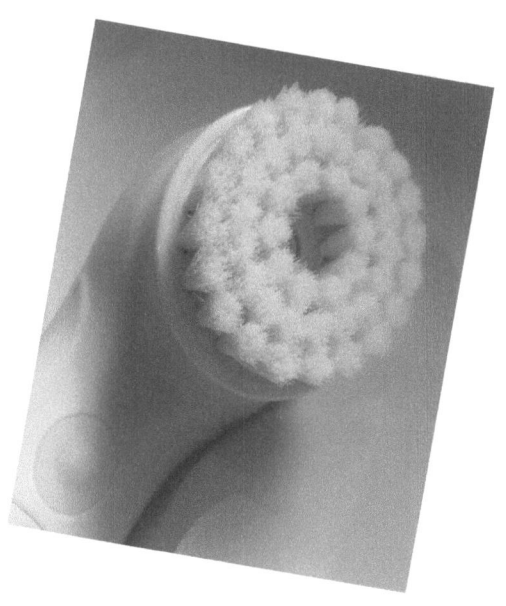

The Benefits on using a Facial brush:

1. It speeds up cell rejuvenation, giving you younger, more vibrant looking skin and reversing the effects of aging.

2. It works by giving you a brighter complexion which looks refreshed rather than gray and dingy. It also improves circulation to the surface of the skin and gives you a rosy glow.

3. Another way it works is by strengthening the skin's structure, giving you softer smoother skin. It does this by removing dead skin and preventing clogged pores. Of course, without doing this treatment, it would lead to blackheads and other skin problems. A big bonus is that your skin will be less prone to breakouts.

Chapter 8   Skin Care for Woman in their 20's

If you are in your 20's, whether just out of your teen years or approaching 30,   there are still specific skin care tips that most of us don't give enough thought to. Graduating college, overcoming self identity issues, and tight budgets create a lot of stress for women in their 20's.

"An ounce of preparation is worth a pound of cure." That statement, all you young women, is of extreme importance to you. The most important way to continue to look great in the years to come and continue with a great glow of youth, is to develop good skin care habits NOW! Almost every woman I know that is over 30 longs for the days of her early 20's.

Those were the years that her skin naturally looked the best. The problem is they didn't take care of themselves and develop the habits that I'm addressing here. Please take this skin care advice, as it will help you tremendously in the years to come. Then you can send me a thank you card.

1. Use sunscreen that is of SPF 35, at least 15 minutes before stepping out into the sun.
2. Find a sunscreen that isn't oily. If you're going to apply make-up, do so after applying the sunscreen, or find make up that has a SPF in it (CC Cream)

3. Splash water on your face a few times during the day if possible, and even in the evening.

4. Wash your face and apply a night cream (that suits your skin type) before going to sleep.

Botanical Products (Go All Natural) could be the option to try for teens and young adult women. Just like women in their 30s and older, the process is the same but with a different kind of product. That product should contain milk thistle, which is a powerful antioxidant that helps defend against environmental damage while helping to calm and soothe skin.

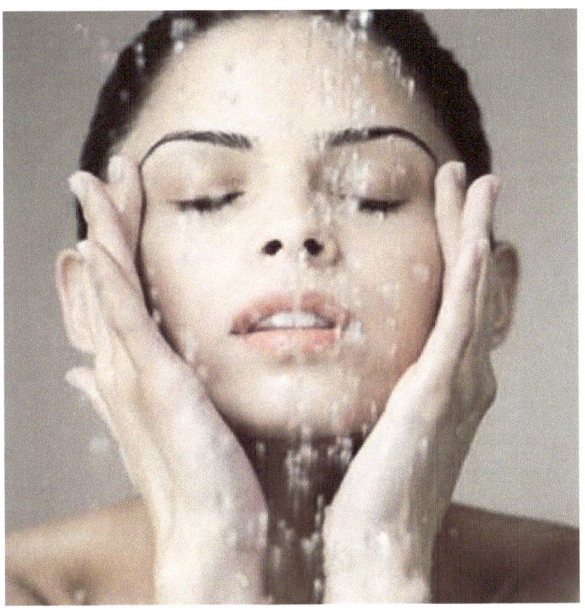

Cleanser -Cleansers help to remove all of the dirt, oil and other impurities from skin. Removing makeup is an absolute must, and even more so as we enter our twenties.

Exfoliate Mask- In addition to daily cleansing, now is the time to kick things up a notch with a good exfoliating scrub. Mask scrubs are essential when it comes to getting rid of those drab, dead skin cells that build up on the surface. Those yucky, dead skin cells can clog our pores and lead to breakouts. We all want to avoid breakouts at any cost, no matter what age.

Refreshing- Cleanse the skin, and refresh and shrink the appearance of pores on the face. Toners can be applied to the skin in different ways; cotton, wool, or spraying them on to the face.

Moisturizing Day & Night- It's essential to make sure your youthful skin has all of the proper hydration that it needs to look and function at its best. Invest in a good facial moisturizer and night cream right away! Never miss an opportunity to moisturize your skin.

Proper hydration will keep your skin looking young and fresh. You may have been able to skip your night creams up until now, but in your 20's, start taking advantage of those products that will deliver benefits to your skin.

Protecting Your skin from Sun- Most skin cancer is caused by sun damage that occurred before the age of 20. Always use a sunscreen or moisturizer that contains an SPF 35,even a CC cream foundation with SPF 35. Re-apply sunscreen frequently. Even though many brands claim to be waterproof, eventually they wear off. That way you will have advance protection, regardless of whether you are in or out of the sun.

Become familiar with the term "Anti-Aging"

Anti-aging products are not just for Mom and Grandma. If you're in your twenties, you need to embrace the term "Anti-Aging". These words are very positive, and will surely become your go-to words in skin care products. Our skin ages at different rates due to many different factors, including our lifestyle. Anti-aging products act as a proactive measure to keep skin looking good. We must put up the good fight against the signs of aging.

Sometimes you just have to be smart. It takes a smart woman to truly think ahead and understand what lies in the future. You just can't avoid the aging process, but as stated above, you can keep it at bay by proper planning an implementation. By doing it now, you will really see the benefits later.

Chapter 9   Skin Care for Women in Their 30's

Sorry to tell you young ladies, but you've moved on to join us "older folks". If you've done your job properly, your 20's skin hasn't changed much. If you didn't use the sunscreen that was really important to keeping that youthful complexion, you have a little work to do. You ladies that basked in the sun are probably starting to see some fine lines, a little elasticity loss, and maybe a few dark spots.

The good news is that it's never too late. Even though this is the time in your life signs of aging may appear (crow's feet, eyelid sagging, some dark circles, a few of the following steps can make a huge difference as to your skin and the way it looks.

Cleansers for Normal to Dry to Oily Skin type

Different types of cleansers have been developed for people with different skin types. Active cleansers are more suitable for oily skins to prevent breakouts. Very dry skin may require a creamy lotion-type cleanser.

These are normally too gentle to be effective on oily or even normal skin, but dry skin requires much less cleansing power. It may be a good idea to select a cleanser that is alcohol-free for use on dry, sensitive, or dehydrated skin.

This helps to unclog pores and prevent skin conditions such as acne. A cleanser can be used as part of a skin care regimen together with a toner and moisturizer.

Did you know that many visible signs of aging on your skin have to do with external causes? So if you're looking to revamp your skin care routine and tighten your skin, start by cleaning up the way you cleanse.

Facial cleanser gets rid of old surface skin cells, dirt, dust, make-up,
and bacteria, and allows your pores to breathe freely. It also helps your circulation and prepares your skin to properly receive any topical products you use.

3 Essential Skin Care Benefits In A Cleanser

There are cleansers that combine age-fighting benefits

1. To Cleanse
2. Exfoliate
3. Refresh - Revealing Younger-Looking Skin.

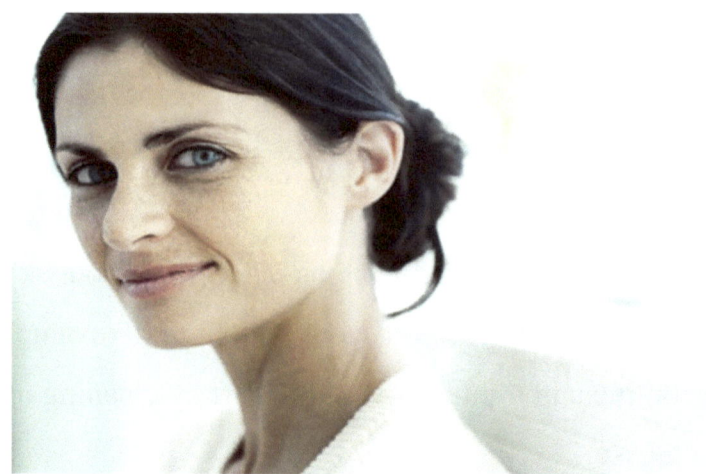

Age-Fighting Moisturizer

The Age-Fighting Moisturizer brings you advanced benefits that are proven to hydrate the skin . Moisturizer lotion absorbs quickly, leaving the skin soft, always fresh, Oil and fragrance-free, and will not clog pores. And the right skin type for your skin. If you are an oily skin type, you should only apply a small portion. Because the skin is already oily too much Moisturizer will create too much shine, which of course you don't want. Age-Fighting Moisturizer will help prevent fine wrinkles and make you look more rejuvenated, looking better than ever.

Sun Screen / Day Solution

Dermatologists believe it's important we all understand the latest research on sun damage and update our sunscreen protection accordingly. Choose a sunscreen that has SPF 35 to help prevent skin cancer.

There are 4 reasons we should use this daily; after our cleanser and before our foundation.

1. Skin cancer rates are on the rise and sunscreen has been proven to help decrease the development of skin cancer.

2. It helps to prevent facial brown spots and skin discolorations.

3. It also helps to reduce the appearance of facial red veins

4. It slows down the development of wrinkled, premature aging skin.

Night Solution

Nighttime is when skin does its heavy lifting. Night Solution skin does the bulk of its repairing, restoring, and regenerating while we sleep, so night creams are focused on moisture and recovery. They contain the most powerful and slow-absorbing moisturizers that are designed to penetrate over the course of several hours. Since there's little to no concern about sun exposure, they also contain the highest concentrations of anti-aging compound ingredients like retinol, glycolic acid, and hyaluronic acid, which are able to do their work without interference from sunscreens.

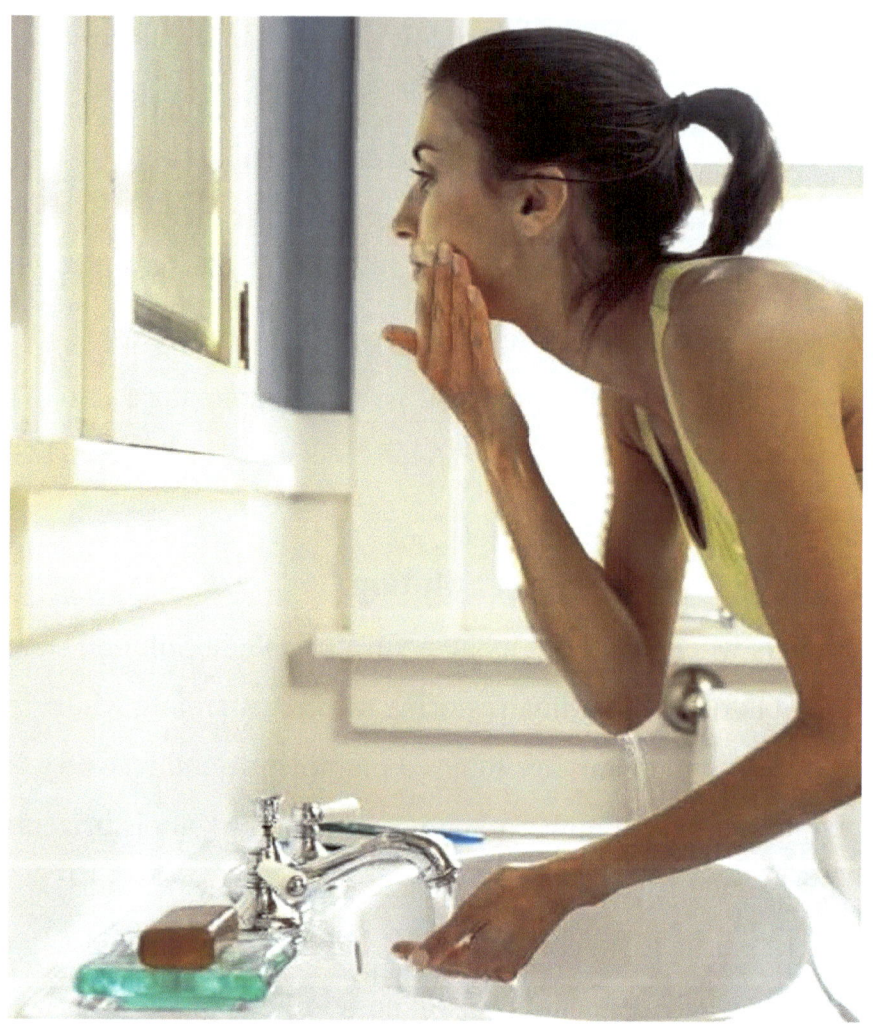

It's obvious that the older you get, the more attention you need to pay to skin care. Women throughout the ages have searched for that "fountain of youth". Today's research and product development has brought many new and innovative skin care treatments for women 30 and older. Utilizing these wonderful methods will give any woman a big edge on keeping that youthful look.

Chapter 10   In Your 40's

Here's the bad news: aging is inevitable. But the good news is you don't need to be blessed with perfect genetics to have youthful, glowing skin, no matter how old you really are. Problems with sun damaged skin continue to grow for fair skinned women, and may show up as dark spots, hyperpigmentation, or splotchiness. For darker complexions, fine lines, wrinkles and loss of volume become much more of an issue. In addition, some specific problems can occur when hormone related issues become apparent, such as acne and dryness caused by pre-menopause.

For women in that age range follow the formulation that I've given below, as that will help you tremendously in your eternal quest for that youthful appearance. Many of these are the same as the 30's application, with a few exceptions.

Topical Products You Use.

Age-Fighting Cleanser For Your Skin Type

Did you know that many visible signs of aging on your skin have to do with external causes? So if you're looking to revamp your skin care routine and tighten your skin, start by cleaning up the way you cleanse.

Facial cleanser gets rid of old surface skin cells, dirt, dust, make-up,
and bacteria, and allows your pores to breathe freely. It also helps your circulation and prepares your skin to properly receive any topical products you use.

3 Essential Skin Care Benefits In A Cleanser

There are cleansers that combine age-fighting benefits

1.To Cleanse

2.Exfoliate

3.Refresh - Revealing Younger-Looking Skin.

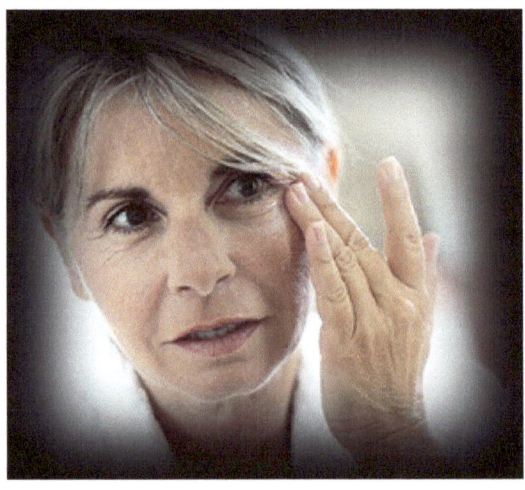

Age-Fighting Moisturizer

The Age-Fighting Moisturizer brings you advanced benefits that are proven to hydrate the skin . Moisturizer lotion absorbs quickly, leaving the skin soft, always fresh, Oil and fragrance-free, and will not clog pores. And the right skin type for your skin. If you are an oily skin type, you should only apply a small portion. Because the skin is already oily too much Moisturizer will create too much shine, which of course you don't want. Age-Fighting Moisturizer will help prevent fine wrinkles and make you look more rejuvenated, looking better than ever.

Sun Screen / Day Solution

Dermatologists believe it's important we all understand the latest research on sun damage and update our sunscreen protection accordingly. Choose a sunscreen that has SPF 35 to help prevent skin cancer. There are 4 reasons we should use this daily; after our cleanser and before our foundation.

1. Skin cancer rates are on the rise and sunscreen has been proven to help decrease the development of skin cancer.
2. It helps to prevent facial brown spots and skin discolorations.
3. It also helps to reduce the appearance of facial red veins
4. It slows down the development of wrinkled, premature aging skin.

Night Solution

Nighttime is when skin does its heavy lifting. Night Solution skin does the bulk of its repairing, restoring, and regenerating while we sleep, so night creams are focused on moisture and recovery. They contain the most powerful and slow-absorbing moisturizers that are designed to penetrate over the course of several hours. Since there's little to no concern about sun exposure, they also contain the highest concentrations of anti-aging compound ingredients like retinol, glycolic acid, and hyaluronic acid, which are able to do their work without interference from sunscreens.

Additional moisturizers and serums to help our age group keep the skin in wonderful condition.

Chapter 11   The 50's and Beyond

Just because you've reached the *WONDER YEARS* doesn't mean that you concede to them. You're a beautiful woman, with many years left to show off that fantastic complexion. So live like it !!! And that can mean following a very specific but relatively simple formula for that complexion we're talking about here.

Living the right way, especially if you've been following that regimen for the previous years, can pave the way for continued success regarding your skin condition. For those of you that have been more tough on your body, you may have a little more difficult time in achieving the desired results, but never fear. It most certainly can be accomplished, and you need to put your mind to it in a way that allows for it to happen. If you smoke, quit. If you love the sun TOO MUCH, cut back and use the necessary sunscreen.

Look, age happens, but you can truly slow it down and sometimes put it on hold. You may be noticing thinner and sagging skin, deepening wrinkles, lines and hyper pigmentation. Maybe the skin has become overly dry and flaky. It just doesn't matter, as long as you are up to the challenge of changing poor habits and becoming attuned to the right methods of achieving that youthful appearance. It can be done.

By utilizing the processes and products that apply to the women in the 40's and adding the following, everything will change for the better. Here's a few extras to get you going:

- The cleanser continues to be of major importance. Age can seriously create additional dryness, and you need to be cognizant of the need to use a creamy moisturizing cleanser to minimize the damage to sensitive skin.

- Antioxidants are extremely important here. And then using a layer of broad-spectrum sunscreen with an SPF 30 will help a bunch. This moisturizing potion will enables the skin to become rejuvenated, and you can feel the difference.

And lastly, using creams with hydroquinone, kojic acid, and phytophenol can truly help reduce hyper pigmentation.

1. Cleanser
2. Microdermabrasion twice a week
3. Facial Mask twice week
4. Moisturizer
5. Day sunscreen SPF 35 / Night solution

Chapter 12 Men Skincare

Some say women are more sensitive than men, and it's definitely true when it comes to your face. Men facial skin is typically thicker than women and less likely to be sensitive to ingredients in facial cleansers and moisturizers. Skincare is also usually a simpler routine since men typically don't wear makeup.

The psychological factor for men comes into play when it comes to skin care. There are those men that appear nonchalant when you talk to them about their skin, but when alone are very attentive to the way their skin appears. And then there are those who take a tremendous pride in their skin, and will do virtually anything to make themselves blemish free. Regardless of the approach of the particular man, there are very specific products and methods to keep the skin healthy and looking great.

Bar Soap or Liquid Cleansers for Men

Most men prefer bars soap than liquid cleansers. That's fine as long as they have normal or oily skin. But bar soap tends to dry skin out more than liquid cleansers. If your skin feels tight or a little itchy after you wash your face, try switching to a liquid cleanser.

1. But if you insist on using a bar soap, look for moisturizing soaps with emollients such as glycerin.

2. Men may experience problems with acne if they have very oily skin. Acne is caused by excess oil production that clogs pores, causing inflammation.

3. Look for acne treatment that contain salicylic acid, glycolic acid, or benzyl peroxide. All three of these exfoliating agents remove the upper layers of dead skin and allow for deeper cleaning of pores. They also have antibacterial properties.

Moisturizers for Men

To moisten your skin after washing it, you need to apply a moisturizer.

1. For dry skin, choose a cream, which is the thickest formulation.

2. For normal skin, reach for a lotion, which is lighter and less oily.

3. For oily skin, choose a skin toner or gel.

Sunscreen Protection for Men

You'll get far more protection over time by making sure you use a face moisturizer with sunscreen in it every day, moisturizer products with retinol (Retin-A) do smooth out fine lines and wrinkles and even reverse signs of aging at the cellular level.

Shaving Products for Men

Most men find a comfortable way to shave and stick with it. If you're still suffering nicks, cuts, razor burn, or razor bumps, it's time for a change. Try the foam cream that contains, Glycerin, Lanolin, Aloe Leaf Extract, cucumber and Fruit Extract. By using these ingredients, you will greatly alleviate skin irritation.

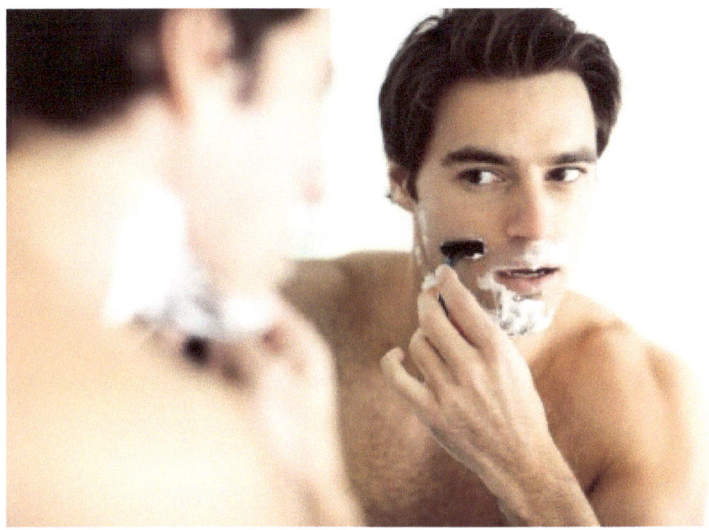

Keeping men updated on the proper methods of skin care can be a daunting task, especially those that that take the nonchalant approach. However, especially for the loved ones in your life, a little push and a lot of information, spoken gently, can greatly assist them in achieving healthy and great looking skin.

Chapter 13 Let's Make You Even More Beautiful

The more women I talk to, the more I realize the incredible need for proper direction in regards to solving their skin issues. For many, it's extremely traumatic, having skin problems that they just don't know how to solve.

Writing this book has enabled me to not only address the needs of those women, but actually educate myself as to the way of getting the message out to those that feel lost. It has become evident that without the proper guidance, women are buying products that just won't help, or are actually working against the efforts to have beautiful skin.

My main goal has become pretty simple. Find a way to deliver the right message out to those lost women, and enable them to actually change their life's. Because having that beautiful skin does change their life. It's not just a matter of beauty either. It's a matter of health when you take care of the skin in the proper way, you are taking care of your body.And to teach women how to strive in a successful way to achieve their goals and to try something different in life.

And here's the wonder of the whole thing. Once you start to look better, you feel better and you will be a happier person. And once that glows out to the whole world, those around you will recognize it and it will be a WOW !! Moment for everyone around you. It's a truly remarkable cycle.

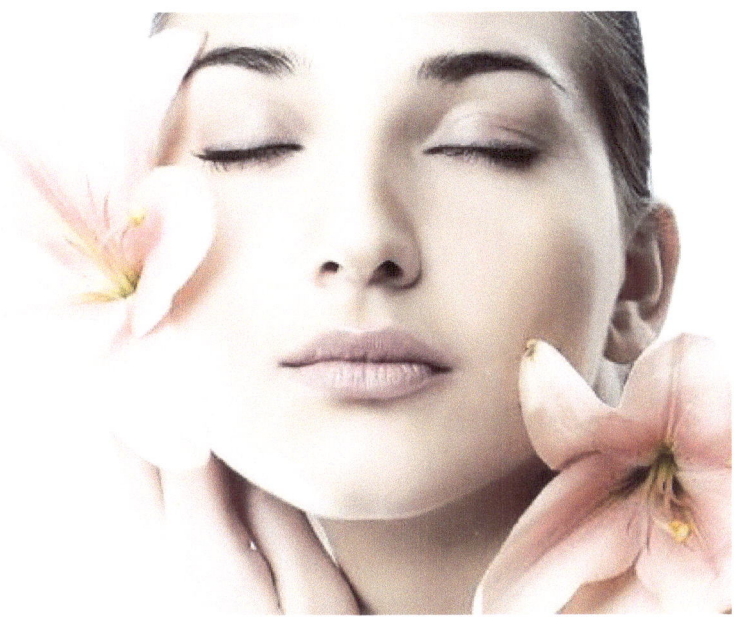

My door is open to you. It's extremely simple throughout the book I've given you various ways to contact me.So are you ready to get glowing and have a beautiful skin complexion ? Your call !!! I thank you for having the time in reading this book and hope to keep providing you with the BEST of my Beauty tips.Hope to here from you we'll talk soon..